Super Fast Comfort Food Recipes for Busy People

Busy People

The definitive delicious comfort food collection for everyday

Jerry Fraction

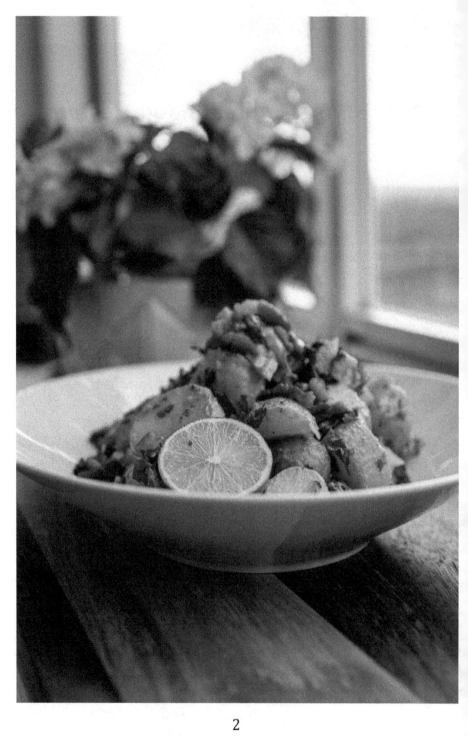

professional advice. The content within this book has been derived from various sources. Please consult a licensed professional before attempting any techniques outlined in this book.

By reading this document, the reader agrees that under no circumstances is the author responsible for any losses, direct or indirect, which are incurred as a result of the use of information contained within this document, including, but not limited to, — errors, omissions, or inaccuracies.

Table of Contents

Salmon and Artichokes

Preparation time: 10 minutes | Cooking Time: 15 minutes | Servings: 4

Ingredients:

1-pound salmon, skinless, boneless, and cubed

2 spring onions, chopped

12 ounces canned artichokes, roughly chopped

1 and ½ cups chicken stock

A pinch of salt and black pepper

1 tablespoon cilantro, chopped

Directions:

In your Pressure Pot, combine all the ingredients, put the lid on, and cook on High for 15 minutes.

Release the pressure naturally for 10 minutes, divide everything between plates and serve.

Nutrition:

Calories 193, fat 7.1g, fiber 4.1g, carbs 6.4g, protein 24.5g.

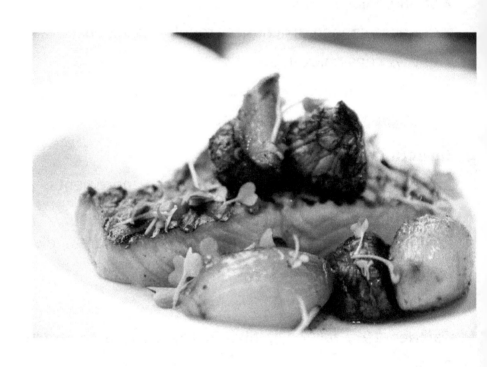

Trout and Spinach Mix

Preparation time: 5 minutes | Cooking Time: 15 minutes | Servings: 4

Ingredients:

6 trout fillets, boneless

2 tablespoons avocado oil

2 scallions, minced

2 garlic cloves, minced

2 tablespoons cilantro, chopped

1 cup baby spinach

A pinch of salt and black pepper

2 tablespoons balsamic vinegar

Directions:

Set the Pressure Pot on Sauté mode, add the oil, heat it, add the scallions and the garlic and sauté for 2 minutes.

Add the rest of the ingredients, put the lid on, and cook on High for 12 minutes.

Release the pressure fast for 5 minutes, divide the mix between plates and serve.

Nutrition:

Calories 194, fat 8.8g, fiber 0.7g, carbs 1.8g, protein 25.4g.

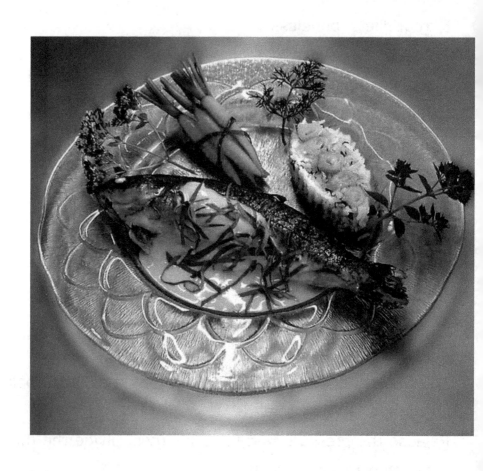

Sea Bass and Sauce

Preparation time: 10 minutes | Cooking Time: 15 minutes | Servings: 4

Ingredients:

4 sea bass fillets, boneless and skinless

2 tablespoons lime juice

2 garlic cloves, minced

1 shallot, chopped

1 cup chicken stock

1 cup tomato passata

A pinch of salt and black pepper

Directions:

In your Pressure Pot, combine the fish with the rest of the ingredients, put the lid on, and cook on High for 15 minutes.

Release the pressure naturally for 10 minutes, divide the mix between plates and serve.

Nutrition:

Calories 154, fat 2.9g, fiber 1.3g, carbs 2.5g, protein 25g.

Sea Bass and Pesto

Preparation time: 5 minutes | Cooking Time: 12 minutes | Servings: 4

Ingredients:

4 sea bass fillets, skinless, boneless

2 tablespoons olive oil

2 tablespoons garlic, chopped

1 cup basil, chopped

2 tablespoons pine nuts

A pinch of salt and black pepper

1 cup tomato passata

1 tablespoon parsley, chopped

Directions:

In your blender, combine the oil with the garlic, basil, pine nuts, salt, and pepper and pulse well.

In your Pressure Pot, combine the sea bass with the pesto, salt, pepper, tomato passata, and parsley, put the lid on, and cook on High for 12 minutes.

Release the pressure fast for 5 minutes, divide the mix between plates and serve.

Nutrition:

Calories 237, fat 12.7g, fiber 1.3g, carbs 5.5g, protein 25.8g.

Tuna and Mustard Greens

Preparation time: 10 minutes | Cooking Time: 10 minutes | Servings: 4

Ingredients:

2 cups mustard greens

1 tablespoon olive oil

1 cup tomato passata

1 shallot, chopped

1 tablespoon basil, chopped

A pinch of salt and black pepper

14 ounces tuna fillets, boneless, skinless, and cubed

Directions:

Set your Pressure Pot on Sauté mode, add the oil, heat it, add the shallot and sauté for 2 minutes.

Add rest of the ingredients, put the lid on, and cook on High for 8 minutes.

Release the pressure naturally for 10 minutes, divide the mix between plates and serve.

Nutrition:

Calories 124g, fat 3.7g, fiber 1.9g, carbs 2.6g, protein 1.6g.

Salmon and Salsa

Preparation time: 10 minutes | Cooking Time: 8 minutes | Servings: 4

Ingredients:

4 salmon fillets, boneless

½ cup veggie stock

1 cup black olives, pitted

1 cup tomatoes, cubed

1 tablespoon basil, chopped

1 tablespoon olive oil

1 tablespoon balsamic vinegar

A pinch of salt and black pepper

1 tablespoon chives, chopped

Directions:

In your Pressure Pot, combine the fish with the stock, salt, and pepper put the lid on, and cook on High for 8 minutes.

Release the pressure naturally for 10 minutes and divide the salmon between plates.

In a bowl, mix the olives with the rest of the ingredients, toss, add next to the salmon and serve.

Nutrition:

Calories 313, fat 18.2g, fiber 1.7g, carbs 4g, protein 35.4g.

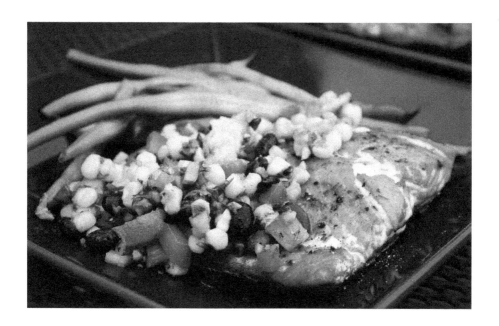

Tex-Mex Chicken Casserole

Preparation Time: 10 minutes | Cooking Time: 30 minutes | Servings: 4

Ingredients:

4 cups cooked chicken, shredded

1/2 cup can corn, drained

2 tbsp milk

2 tbsp taco seasoning

10 oz can cream of chicken soup

2 cups Colby jack cheese, grated

1 cup instant rice

10 oz can Rotel

Directions:

Spray Pressure Pot from inside with cooking spray.

Add all ingredients except 1/2 cup Colby jack cheese into the Pressure Pot and stir until well combined.

Sprinkle 1/2 cup Colby jack cheese on top.

Seal pot with air fryer lid and select bake mode then set the temperature to 350° F and timer for 30 minutes.

Serve and enjoy.

Nutrition:

Calories 945, Fat 27.8g, Carbs 110.5g, Sugar 2.9g, Protein 60.6g, Cholesterol 165mg.

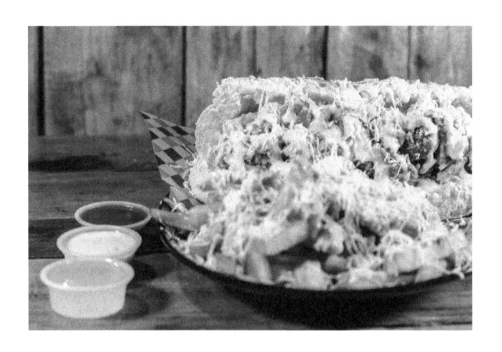

Parmesan Flank Steak

Preparation Time: 10 minutes | Cooking Time: 12 minutes | Servings: 2

Ingredients:

1 lb flank steak

2 tbsp parmesan cheese, grated

2 tbsp olive oil

Pepper

Salt

Directions:

Coat steak with oil and season with pepper and salt.

Sprinkle parmesan cheese on top of the steak.

Place the dehydrating tray in a multi-level air fryer basket and place basket in the Pressure Pot.

Place steak on dehydrating tray.

Seal pot with air fryer lid and select air fry mode then set the temperature to 400° F and timer for 12 minutes.

Turn steak halfway through.

Serve and enjoy.

Nutrition:

Calories 578, Fat 34.1g, Carbohydrates 0.2g, Sugar 0g, Protein 64.9g, Cholesterol 129mg.

Cranberry Meatballs

Preparation Time: 10 minutes | Cooking Time: 5 minutes | Servings: 2

Ingredients:

14 oz frozen meatballs

6 oz chili sauce

7 oz jelly cranberry sauce

Directions:

Place the dehydrating tray in a multi-level air fryer basket and place basket in the Pressure Pot.

Place meatballs on a dehydrating tray.

Seal pot with air fryer lid and select air fry mode then set the temperature to 350° F and timer for 5 minutes.

Meanwhile, in a mixing bowl mix together chili sauce and cranberry sauce.

Add meatballs and toss well to coat.

Serve and enjoy.

Nutrition:

Calories 643, Fat 35.5g, Carbohydrates 47g, Sugar 33.4g, Protein 28.1g, Cholesterol 113mg.

Hamburger Cheese Pasta

Preparation Time: 10 minutes | Cooking Time: 8 minutes | Servings: 6

Ingredients:

1 lb ground beef

8 oz milk

1 tbsp garlic powder

1 tbsp onion powder

1 cup cheddar cheese, shredded

8 oz Velveeta cheese, cut into cubes

2 cups chicken broth

16 oz elbow pasta

Directions:

Add the meat into the Pressure Pot and cook on sauté mode until browned. Turn off Pressure Pot.

Add noodles, milk, garlic powder, onion powder, and broth and stir well.

Seal the pot with a pressure-cooking lid and cook on high pressure for 4 minutes.

Once done, release pressure using quick release. Open the lid.

Sprinkle cheddar cheese and Velveeta cheese on top.

Seal pot with air fryer lid and select broil mode then set the timer for 4 minutes.

Serve and enjoy.

Nutrition:

Calories 648, Fat 21.6g, Carbs 65.1g, Sugar 8.2g, Protein 47.1g, Cholesterol 117mg.

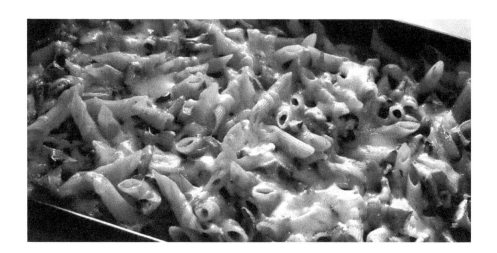

Easy Tuna Casserole

Preparation Time: 10 minutes | Cooking Time: 8 minutes | Servings: 6

Ingredients:

4 cups cooked egg noodles

1 1/2 cups cheddar cheese, shredded

1 cup milk

8 oz cream cheese, softened

1 cup green peas

9 oz can tuna, shredded

8 oz mushrooms, sliced

1 small onion, diced

2 tbsp olive oil

Directions:

Add olive oil into the Pressure Pot and set the pot on sauté mode.

Add onion and mushrooms and sauté until onion is softened. Turn off the sauté mode.

Add egg noodles, 1 cup cheese, milk, cream cheese, green peas, and tuna, and stir well.

Sprinkle remaining cheese on top.

Seal pot with air fryer lid and select bake mode then set the temperature to 375° F and timer for 15 minutes.

Serve and enjoy.

Nutrition:

Calories 535, Fat 30.8g, Carbohydrates 36g, Sugar 5g, Protein 29.5g, Cholesterol 118mg.

Classic Salsa Taco Pasta

Preparation Time: 10 minutes | Cooking Time: 8 minutes | Servings: 6

Ingredients:

1 lb ground beef

1 packet taco seasoning

16 oz cheddar cheese, shredded

32 oz salsa

1 tsp ground cumin

1 tsp garlic powder

1 tbsp hot sauce

2 cups chicken broth

16 oz elbow macaroni

Pepper

Salt

Directions:

Add meat, garlic powder, and cumin into the Pressure Pot and cook on sauté mode until meat is browned.

Add remaining ingredients except for cheese and stir well.

Seal the pot with a pressure-cooking lid and cook on high pressure for 4 minutes.

Once done, release pressure using quick release. Remove lid.

Sprinkle cheese on top.

Seal pot with air fryer lid and select broil mode then set the timer for 4 minutes.

Serve and enjoy.

Nutrition:

Calories 795, Fat 32.4g, Carbohydrates 68.6g, Sugar 7.4g, Protein 56.4g, Cholesterol 149mg.

Spicy Sausage Pasta

Preparation Time: 10 minutes | Cooking Time: 14 minutes | Servings: 4

Ingredients:

1 lb smoked sausage, sliced

1 cup cheddar cheese, shredded

8 oz penne pasta

1/2 cup heavy cream

10 oz can Rotel

2 cups chicken broth

1 tsp garlic, minced

1/2 onion, diced

1 tbsp olive oil

Pepper

Salt

Directions:

Add olive oil into the Pressure Pot and set the pot on sauté mode.

Add garlic, onion, and sausage and sauté until onion is softened about 5 minutes.

Add cream, tomatoes, broth, pasta, pepper, and salt and stir well.

Seal the pot with a pressure-cooking lid and cook on high pressure for 5 minutes.

Once done, release pressure using quick release. Remove lid.

Sprinkle cheese on top.

Seal pot with air fryer lid and select broil mode then set the timer for 4 minutes.

Serve and enjoy.

Nutrition:

Calories 1030, Fat 53.8g, Carbohydrates 86g, Sugar 3.6g, Protein 47.1g, Cholesterol 187mg.

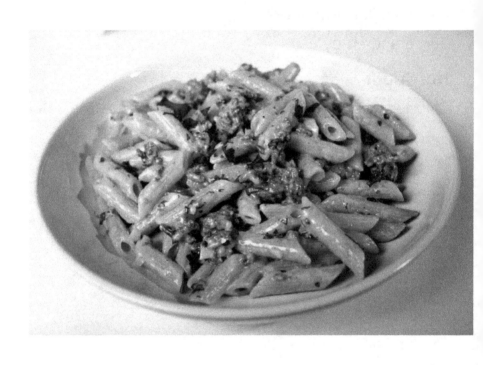

Parmesan Chicken Casserole

Preparation Time: 10 minutes | Cooking Time: 45 minutes | Servings: 6

Ingredients:

2 lbs chicken breasts, boneless and cut into bite-size piece

5 oz garlic croutons, crushed

1/2 cup parmesan cheese, shredded

3 cups mozzarella cheese, shredded

25 oz jar marinara sauce

1/4 cup basil, chopped

1/4 tsp red pepper flakes

2 garlic cloves, minced

Directions:

Spray Pressure Pot from inside with cooking spray.

Add chicken into the Pressure Pot and season with basil, red pepper flakes, and garlic.

Pour the marinara sauce on top of the chicken. sprinkle 1/2 parmesan cheese and half mozzarella cheese on top of the sauce.

Sprinkle crushed croutons then remaining cheeses on top.

Seal pot with air fryer lid and select bake mode then set the temperature to 350° F and timer for 45 minutes. Serve and enjoy.

Nutrition:

Calories 523, Fat 20.8g, Carbohydrates 27.7g, Sugar 5.8g, Protein 53.6g, Cholesterol 147mg.

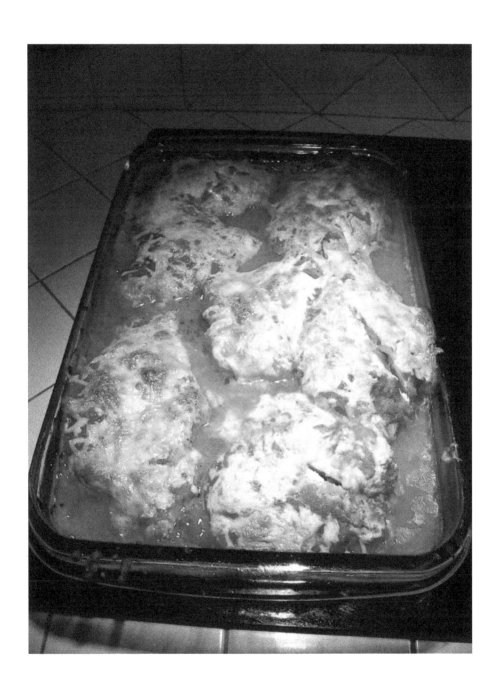

Cauliflower Casserole

Preparation Time: 10 minutes | Cooking Time: 35 minutes | Servings: 6

Ingredients:

1 cauliflower head, cut into florets

1 1/2 cups cheddar cheese, shredded

1 cup milk

3 tbsp all-purpose flour

3 tbsp butter

1 cup of corn

Pepper

Salt

Directions:

Add cauliflower florets into boiling water and boil for 5 minutes. Drain well and set aside.

Add butter into the Pressure Pot and set the pot on sauté mode.

Add flour and stir until smooth. Add 1/2 cup cheese and milk and stir until sauce thickens. Turn off the sauté mode.

Add corn and cauliflower and stir until well coated.

Sprinkle remaining cheese on top and season with pepper and salt.

Seal pot with air fryer lid and select bake mode then set the temperature to 350° F and timer for 30 minutes. Serve and enjoy.

Nutrition:

Calories 232, Fat 16.3g, Carbohydrates 12.5g, Sugar 3.9g, Protein 10.5g, Cholesterol 48mg.

Delicious Pesto Salmon

Preparation Time: 10 minutes | Cooking Time: 20 minutes | Servings: 2

Ingredients:

2 salmon fillets

1/4 cup parmesan cheese, grated

For pesto:

1/4 cup olive oil

1 1/2 cups fresh basil leaves

3 garlic cloves, peeled and chopped

1/4 cup parmesan cheese, grated

1/4 cup pine nuts

1/4 tsp black pepper

1/2 tsp salt

Directions:

Add all pesto ingredients into the blender and blend until smooth.

Line Pressure Pot air fryer basket with parchment paper.

Place salmon fillet on parchment paper in the air fryer basket. Spread 2 tablespoons of the pesto on each salmon fillet.

Sprinkle cheese on top of the pesto.

Place basket in the pot.

Seal the pot with an air fryer lid and select bake mode and cook at 400° F for 20 minutes.

Serve and enjoy.

Nutrition:

Calories 589, Fat 48.7g, Carbohydrates 4.5g, Sugar 0.7g, Protein 38.9g, Cholesterol 81mg.

Crisp & Delicious Catfish

Preparation Time: 10 minutes | Cooking Time: 20 minutes | Servings: 2

Ingredients:

2 catfish fillets

1/4 cup cornmeal

1/2 tsp garlic powder

1/2 tsp onion powder

1/2 tsp salt

Directions:

Add cornmeal, garlic powder, onion powder, and salt into a zip-lock bag.

Add fish fillets to the zip-lock bag. Seal bag and shake gently to coat fish fillet.

Line Pressure Pot air fryer basket with parchment paper.

Place coated fish fillets on parchment paper in the air fryer basket. Place basket in the pot.

Seal the pot with an air fryer lid and select air fry mode and cook at 400° F for 20 minutes. Turn fish fillets halfway through.

Serve and enjoy.

Nutrition:

Calories 276, Fat 12.7g, Carbohydrates 12.7g, Sugar 0.5g, Protein 26.3g, Cholesterol 75mg.

Easy Paprika Salmon

Preparation Time: 10 minutes | Cooking Time: 7 minutes | Servings: 2

Ingredients:

2 salmon fillets, remove any bones

2 tsp paprika

2 tsp olive oil

Pepper

Salt

Directions:

Brush each salmon fillet with oil, paprika, pepper, and salt.

Line Pressure Pot air fryer basket with parchment paper.

Place salmon fillets on parchment paper in the air fryer basket. Place basket in the pot.

Seal the pot with an air fryer lid and select air fry mode and cook at 390° F for 7 minutes.

Serve and enjoy.

Nutrition:

Calories 282, Fat 15.9g, Carbohydrates 1.2g, Sugar 0.2g, Protein 34.9g, Cholesterol 78mg.

Ranch Fish Fillets

Preparation Time: 10 minutes | Cooking Time: 12 minutes | Servings: 2

Ingredients:

2 fish fillets

1 egg, lightly beaten

1 1/4 tbsp olive oil

1/4 cup breadcrumbs

1/2 packet ranch dressing mix

Directions:

In a shallow dish, mix breadcrumbs, ranch dressing mix, and oil.

Dip fish fillet in egg then coats with breadcrumb mixture and place on parchment paper in the air fryer basket. Place basket in the pot.

Seal the pot with an air fryer lid and select air fry mode and cook at 400° F for 12 minutes.

Serve and enjoy.

Nutrition:

Calories 373, Fat 22.9g, Carbohydrates 25.7g, Sugar 1.2g, Protein 18g, Cholesterol 113mg.

Crispy Coconut Shrimp

Preparation Time: 10 minutes | Cooking Time: 10 minutes | Servings: 2

Ingredients:

1 cup egg white, lightly beaten

12 large shrimp

1 tbsp cornstarch

1 cup shredded coconut

1 cup flour

1 cup breadcrumbs

Directions:

Line Pressure Pot air fryer basket with parchment paper.

In a shallow dish, mix coconut and breadcrumbs.

In another dish, mix flour and cornstarch.

Add the egg white to a small bowl.

Dip shrimp in egg white then roll in flour mixture and coat with breadcrumb mixture.

Place coated shrimp in an Pressure Pot air fryer basket.

Place basket in the pot.

Seal the pot with an air fryer lid and select air fry mode and cook at 350° F for 10 minutes.

Serve and enjoy.

Nutrition:

Calories 700, Fat 17.6g, Carbs 97.7g, Sugar 6.9g, Protein 35.8g, Cholesterol 69mg.

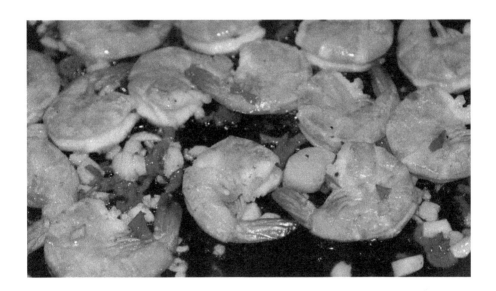

Healthy Shrimp Pasta

Preparation Time: 10 minutes | Cooking Time: 4 minutes | Servings: 6

Ingredients:

1 lb jumbo shrimp, peeled and deveined

1/2 cup green onion, chopped

1 tbsp sriracha sauce

1 1/2 cups yogurt

1 tbsp vinegar

1 lime juice

1/4 cup Fresno pepper, diced

1/4 cup honey

1 tsp coconut oil

1 tsp garlic, minced

4 cups of water

13 oz spaghetti noodles, break in half

1/4 tsp pepper

Directions:

Add oil into the inner pot of Pressure Pot duo crisp and set pot on sauté mode.

Add Fresno peppers and garlic and sauté for 30 seconds.

Add noodles then pour water over noodles.

Add shrimp, lime juice, honey, vinegar, and pepper on top of noodles.

Seal the pot with a pressure-cooking lid and cook on high for 3 minutes.

Once done, release pressure using a quick release. Remove lid.

Add sriracha, yogurt, and green onions and stir well.

Serve and enjoy.

Nutrition:

Calories 348, Fat 4.6g, Carbohydrates 51.5g, Sugar 17.9g, Protein 24.2g, Cholesterol 205mg.

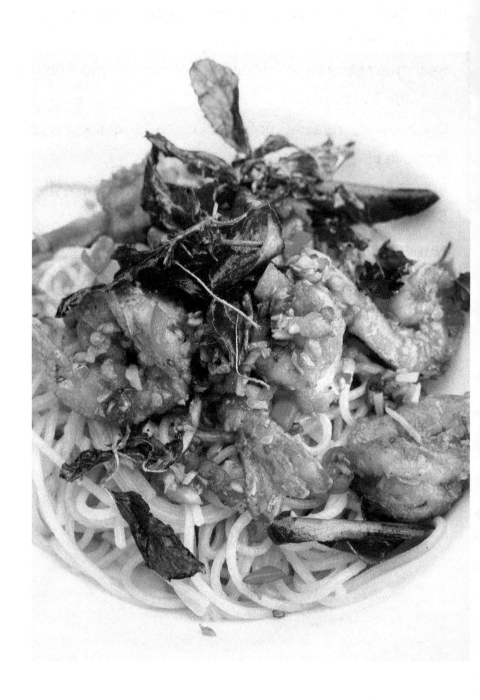

Delicious Cod Nuggets

Preparation Time: 10 minutes | Cooking Time: 15 minutes | Servings: 4

Ingredients:

1 lb cod fillet, cut into chunks

1/2 cup all-purpose flour

1 tbsp olive oil

1 cup cracker crumbs

1 egg, lightly beaten

Pepper

Salt

Directions:

Line Pressure Pot air fryer basket with parchment paper.

Add crackers crumb and oil in the food processor and process until it forms crumbly.

Season fish chunks with pepper and salt.

Coat fish chunks with flour then dip in egg and coat with cracker crumbs.

Place coated fish chunks on parchment paper in the air fryer basket. Place basket in the pot.

Seal the pot with an air fryer lid and select air fry mode and cook at 350° F for 15 minutes.

Serve and enjoy.

Nutrition:

Calories 272, Fat 9.7g, Carbohydrates 21.5g, Sugar 0.4g, Protein 24.4g, Cholesterol 97mg.

Balsamic Salmon

Preparation Time: 10 minutes | Cooking Time: 8 minutes | Servings: 2

Ingredients:

2 salmon fillets

2 tbsp balsamic vinegar

2 tbsp honey

1 cup of water

Pepper

Salt

Directions:

Season salmon with pepper and salt.

In a small bowl, mix vinegar and honey.

Brush salmon with vinegar and honey mixture.

Pour water into the inner pot of Pressure Pot duo crisp then place steamer rack into the pot.

Place salmon skin-side down on the steamer rack.

Seal the pot with a pressure-cooking lid and cook on high for 3 minutes.

Once done, release pressure using a quick release. Remove lid.

Seal the pot with an air fryer lid and select air fry mode and cook at 400° F for 5 minutes.

Serve and enjoy.

Nutrition:

Calories 303, Fat 11g, Carbohydrates 17.5g, Sugar 17.3g, Protein 34.6g, Cholesterol 78mg.

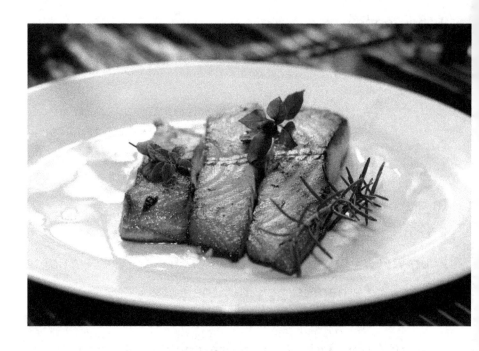

Garlic Shrimp

Preparation Time: 10 minutes | Cooking Time: 8 minutes | Servings: 4

Ingredients:

1 lb shrimp, peeled and deveined

2 tsp olive oil

For sauce:

1/4 cup honey

1/4 cup soy sauce

1 tbsp ginger, minced

1 tbsp garlic, minced

Directions:

In a mixing bowl, mix all sauce ingredients. Add shrimp into the bowl and toss well.

Add oil, shrimp with sauce mixture into the inner pot of Pressure Pot duo crisp and cook on sauté mode for 3 minutes.

Seal the pot with a pressure-cooking lid and cook on high for 5 minutes.

Once done, release pressure using a quick release. Remove lid.

Stir well and serve.

Nutrition:

Calories 235, Fat 4.4g, Carbohydrates 22g, Sugar 17.7g, Protein 27.1g, Cholesterol 239mg.

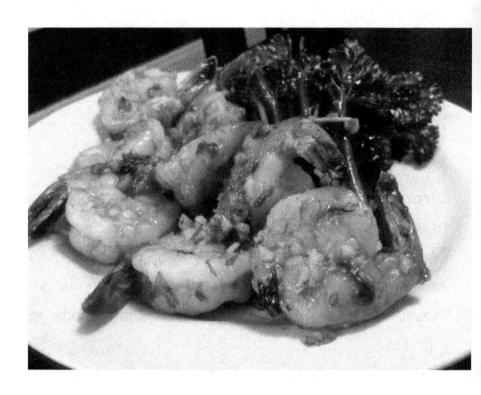

Tuna Noodles

Preparation Time: 10 minutes | Cooking Time: 4 minutes | Servings: 4

Ingredients:

1 can tuna, drained

15 oz egg noodles

3 cups of water

3/4 cup frozen peas

4 oz cheddar cheese, shredded

28 oz can cream of mushroom soup

Directions:

Add noodles and water into the inner pot of Pressure Pot duo crisp and stir well.

Add cream of mushroom soup, peas, and tuna on top of noodles.

Seal the pot with a pressure-cooking lid and cook on high for 4 minutes.

Once done, release pressure using a quick release. Remove lid.

Add cheese and stir well and serve.

Nutrition:

Calories 470, Fat 18.6g, Carbohydrates 47.5g, Sugar 6.2g, Protein 27.7g, Cholesterol 80mg.

Shrimp Scampi

Preparation Time: 10 minutes | Cooking Time: 4 minutes | Servings: 6

Ingredients:

1 lb frozen shrimp

2 cups pasta, uncooked

1/2 tsp paprika

1/2 tsp red pepper flakes

1 tbsp garlic, minced

1/2 cup parmesan cheese

1/2 cup half and half

1 cup chicken broth

2 tbsp butter, melted

Pepper

Salt

Directions:

Add butter into the inner pot of Pressure Pot duo crisp and set pot on sauté mode.

Add garlic, and red pepper flakes and cook for 2 minutes.

Add shrimp, pepper, noodles, paprika, broth, and salt. Stir well.

Seal the pot with a pressure-cooking lid and cook on high for 2 minutes.

Once done, release pressure using a quick release. Remove lid.

Add cheese and half and a half and stir until cheese is melted.

Serve and enjoy.

Nutrition:

Calories 280, Fat 9.3g, Carbohydrates 25.8g, Sugar 0.2g, Protein 22.6g, Cholesterol 164mg.

Greek Burgers

Preparation Time: 10 minutes | Cooking Time: 10 minutes | Servings: 4

Ingredients:

1 1/2 lbs ground beef

1 tsp garlic, minced

1 tbsp fresh lemon juice

1 tbsp oregano

1/2 cup feta cheese, crumbled

Pepper

Salt

Directions:

Add all ingredients into the large bowl and mix until well combined.

Place the dehydrating tray in a multi-level air fryer basket and place basket in the Pressure Pot.

Make four patties from the meat mixture and place them on a dehydrating tray.

Seal pot with air fryer lid and select air fry mode then set the temperature to 380° F and timer for 10 minutes.

Turn patties halfway through.

Serve and enjoy.

Nutrition:

Calories 371, Fat 14.7g, Carbohydrates 1.8g, Sugar 0.9g, Protein 54.5g, Cholesterol 169mg.

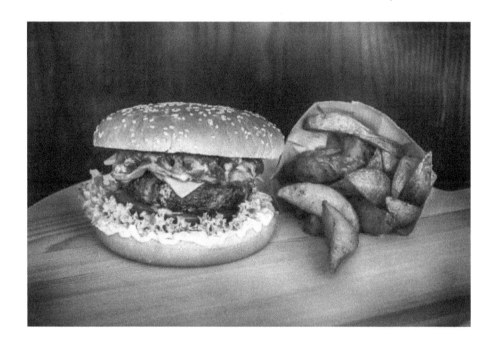

Crispy Honey Garlic Chicken Wings

Preparation time: 10 minutes | Cooking Time: 25 minutes | Servings: 8

Ingredients:

1/8 c. Water

½ tsp. Salt

4 tbsp. Minced garlic

¼ c. Vegan butter

¼ c. Raw honey

¾ c. Almond flour

16 chicken wings

Directions:

Preparing the ingredients. Rinse off and dry chicken wings well.

Spray an instant crisp air fryer basket with olive oil.

Coat chicken wings with almond flour and add coated wings to an instant crisp air fryer.

Air frying. Set temperature to 380°f, and set time to 25 minutes. Cook shaking every 5 minutes.

When the timer goes off, cook 5-10 minutes at 400°f till the skin becomes crispy and dry.

As chicken cooks, melt butter in a saucepan and add garlic. Sauté garlic 5 minutes.

Add salt and honey, simmer for 20 minutes.

Make sure to stir every so often, so the sauce does not burn.

Add a bit of water after 15 minutes to ensure the sauce does not harden.

Take out chicken wings from an instant crisp air fryer and coat in sauce. Enjoy!

Nutrition:

Calories 435, Fat 19g, Protein 31g, Sugar 6g.

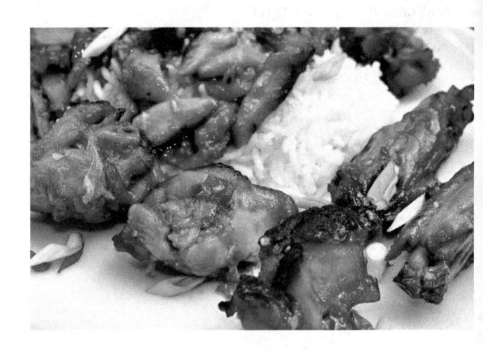

Garlic Basil Carrots

Preparation Time: 10 minutes | Cooking Time: 20 minutes | Servings: 4

Ingredients:

15 baby carrots

6 garlic cloves, minced

4 tbsp olive oil

1 tbsp fresh parsley, chopped

1 tbsp dried basil

1 1/2 tsp salt

Directions:

In a bowl, toss together with oil, carrots, basil, garlic, and salt.

Spray Pressure Pot multi-level air fryer basket with cooking spray.

Transfer carrots into the air fryer basket and place basket into the Pressure Pot.

Seal pot with air fryer lid and select air fry mode then set the temperature to 350°f and timer for 20 minutes. Stir halfway through.

Garnish with parsley and serve.

Nutrition:

Calories 140, Fat 14.1g, Carbohydrates 4.7g, Sugar 1.9g, Protein 0.6g, Cholesterol 0mg.

Italian Seasoned Cauliflower

Preparation Time: 10 minutes | Cooking Time: 12 minutes | Servings: 4

Ingredients:

1 cauliflower head, cut into florets

1/2 tsp Italian seasoning

1/2 tsp garlic powder

1 lemon zest

3 tbsp olive oil

2 tsp lemon juice

1/4 tsp pepper

1/4 tsp salt

Directions:

In a bowl, mix olive oil, lemon juice, Italian seasoning, garlic powder, lemon zest, pepper, and salt.

Add cauliflower florets into the bowl and toss well.

Spray Pressure Pot multi-level air fryer basket with cooking spray.

Add cauliflower florets into the air fryer basket and place basket into the Pressure Pot.

Seal pot with air fryer lid and select air fry mode then set the temperature to 400° F and timer for 12 minutes. Stir halfway through.

Serve and enjoy.

Nutrition:

Calories 115, Fat 10.8g, Carbohydrates 5.3g, Sugar 2.1g, Protein 1.6g, Cholesterol 0mg.

Yummy Chicken Tikka Bites

Preparation Time: 10 minutes | Cooking Time: 12 minutes | Servings: 4

Ingredients:

1 lb chicken breasts, boneless and cut into cubes

1 lemon juice

2 tbsp ghee

1/4 tsp cayenne

1/2 tsp paprika

1/2 tsp ground coriander

1/2 tsp ground cumin

1/2 tsp turmeric

1 tsp garam masala

1/4 cup cilantro, chopped

2 tsp ginger, minced

2 garlic cloves, minced

1/2 cup yogurt

1 tsp salt

Directions:

Add chicken into the mixing bowl.

Pour remaining ingredients over chicken and mix well.

Cover and place in the refrigerator overnight.

Place the dehydrating tray in a multi-level air fryer basket and place basket in the Pressure Pot.

Arrange marinated chicken pieces and place them on a dehydrating tray.

Seal pot with air fryer lid and select air fry mode then set the temperature to 400° F and timer for 12 minutes.

Serve and enjoy.

Nutrition:

Calories 281, Fat 14.2g, Carbohydrates 0.7g, Sugar 0g, Protein 33g, Cholesterol 116mg.

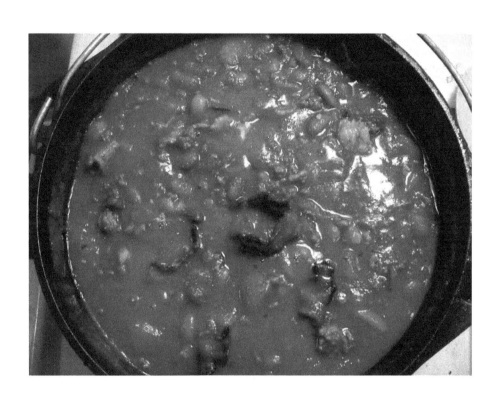

Creamy Mushroom Soup

Preparation Time: 10 minutes | Cooking Time: 10 minutes | Servings: 4

Ingredients:

4 cups mushrooms, sliced

1 tsp dried thyme

3 garlic cloves, minced

1 cup of water

1 jalapeno pepper, chopped

3 cups onion, sliced

1/2 tsp pepper

1 tsp salt

Directions:

Add all ingredients into the Pressure Pot and stir well.

Seal pot with lid and cook on manual high pressure for 10 minutes.

Once done then allow to release pressure naturally for 10 minutes then release using the quick-release method. Open the lid.

Puree the soup using an immersion blender until smooth.

Stir and serve.

Nutrition:

Calories 55, Fat 0.4g, Carbohydrates 11.6g, Sugar 5g, Protein 3.4g, Cholesterol 0mg.

Rosemary Turkey Chowder

Preparation Time: 5 Minutes | Cooking Time: 30 Minutes | Servings:4

Ingredients:

1 ¼ tsp dried Rosemary

2 Celery Stalks, diced

1 cup Broccoli Florets

¾ pound Turkey Breast, cut into cubes

2 tbsp Coconut Oil

½ Yellow Onion, diced

3 ½ cups Homemade Chicken Broth

2/3 pound Sweet Potatoes, cubed

1 tsp minced Garlic

Directions

Set the IP to SAUTE and add the coconut oil to it.

When melted, add the onions and cook for 3 minutes.

Add celery, garlic, and rosemary, and cook for another minute.

Add the turkey cubes and cook until they are no longer brown.

Dump the rest of the ingredients in the IP and stir to combine.

Close the lid and set the Pressure Pot to MANUAL.

Cook on HIGH for 6 minutes.

Do a natural pressure release.

Serve immediately and enjoy!

Nutrition:

Calories 240, Total Fats 12g, Carbs 12g, Protein 28g, Dietary Fiber 2.5g.

Easy Vegetarian Spring Soup

Preparation Time: 5 Minutes | Cooking Time: 25 Minutes | Servings:8

Ingredients:

3 large Carrots, sliced

1 Leek, chopped

8 cups Homemade Bone Broth

2 tsp minced Garlic

4 cups chopped Spinach

10 Radishes, sliced

1 Onion, sliced

1 cup Broccoli Florets

Directions:

Dump all of the ingredients in your Pressure Pot.

Give the mixture a good stir to combine the ingredients well.

Put the lid on and turn it clockwise to seal.

After the chime, press SOUP.

Set the cooking time for 10 minutes.

Let the pressure drop naturally before opening the lid.

Serve immediately.

Enjoy!

Nutrition:

Calories 240, Total Fats 0.2g, Carbs 9g, Protein 20g, Dietary Fiber 2g.

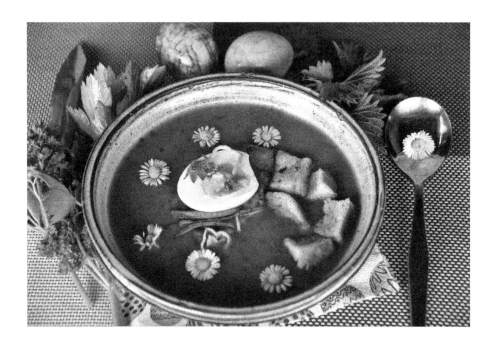

Savory Butternut Squash Soup

Preparation Time: 10 minutes | Cooking Time: 30 minutes | Servings: 8

Ingredients:

6 cups butternut squash, cut into cubes

2 tbsp heavy cream

3 cups vegetable broth

1/4 tsp cinnamon

1 tsp cumin

1 tsp chili powder

2 garlic cloves

1 onion, diced

1/4 tsp pepper

1 tsp kosher salt

Directions:

Add squash, broth, spices, garlic, and onion into the Pressure Pot and stir well.

Seal pot with lid and cook on soup mode for 30 minutes.

Once done then release pressure using the quick-release method then open the lid.

Puree the soup using an immersion blender until smooth.

Add heavy cream and stir well.

Sprinkle chili powder on top of the soup and serve.

Nutrition:

Calories 84, Fat 2.1g, Carbohydrates 14.7g, Sugar 3.2g, Protein 3.3g, Cholesterol 5mg.

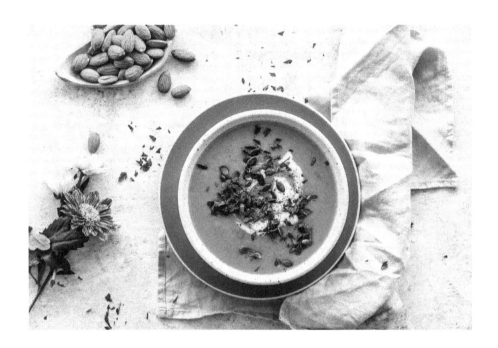

Curried Carrot Soup

Preparation Time: 5 Minutes | Cooking Time: 17 minutes | Servings: 4

Ingredients:

1 1/4 lbs carrot, chopped

1/2 tsp curry powder

1 jalapeno pepper, chopped

1 medium onion, chopped

1/2 cup coconut milk

1/4 tsp cayenne pepper

1/4 tsp turmeric

1/4 tsp garam masala

1 tbsp olive oil

1 tsp garlic powder

1 tsp sea salt

4 cups chicken broth

2 tsp ginger, grated

Directions:

Add oil into the Pressure Pot and set the pot on sauté mode.

Add onion into the pot and sauté for 5 minutes.

Add carrot and pepper and sauté for a minute.

Add remaining ingredients except for coconut milk and stir well.

Seal pot with a lid and select cook on high for 12 minutes.

Release pressure using the quick-release method than open the lid.

Puree the soup using a blender until smooth. Stir in coconut milk.

Serve and enjoy.

Nutrition:

Calories 215, Carbohydrates 20.7g, Protein 7.3 g, Fat 12.2g, Sugar 10.2g, Sodium 1335mg.

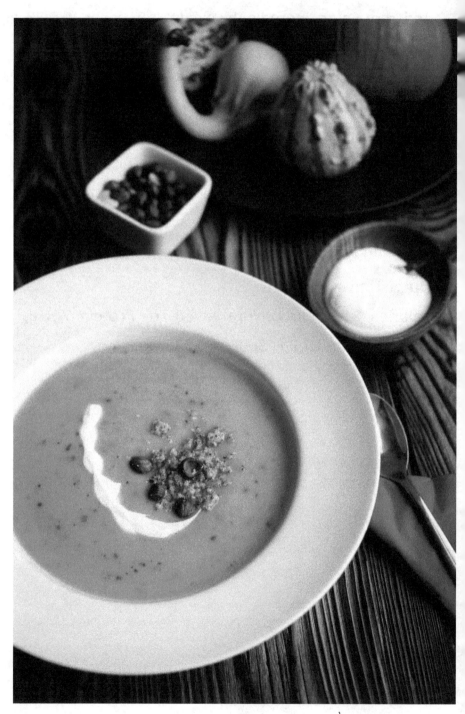

Chicken Celery Soup

Preparation Time: 5 Minutes | Cooking Time: 23 minutes | Servings: 6

Ingredients:

2 chicken breast, skinless and boneless

2 celery stalks, diced

1/2 onion, diced

14 oz coconut milk

4 cups chicken broth

2 carrots, diced

Directions:

Add 1 cup of broth and chicken into the Pressure Pot and stir well.

Seal pot with lid and cook on poultry mode for 8 minutes.

Release pressure using the quick-release method than open the lid.

Add remaining ingredients and stir well.

Again, seal the pot with a lid and cook on soup mode for 15 minutes.

Release pressure using the quick-release method than open the lid.

Serve and enjoy.

Nutrition:

Calories 229, Carbohydrates 7.3g, Protein 12.1g, Fat 17.5g, Sugar 4.1g, Sodium 555mg.

Italian Leek Cabbage Soup

Preparation Time: 5 Minutes | Cooking Time: 20 minutes | Servings: 4

Ingredients:

1/2 cabbage head, chopped

2 tbsp olive oil

2 leeks, chopped

1 garlic clove, minced

2 carrots, diced

1 tsp Creole seasoning

1 tsp Italian seasoning

4 cups chicken broth

1 bell pepper, diced

3 celery ribs, diced

2 cups mixed salad greens

Pepper

Salt

Directions:

Add coconut oil into the Pressure Pot and set the pot on sauté mode.

Add all ingredients except salad greens into the pot and stir well.

Seal pot with lid and cook on soup mode for 20 minutes.

Release pressure using the quick-release method than open the lid.

Add salad greens and stir until it wilts.

Serve and enjoy.

Nutrition:

Calories 191, Carbohydrates 21.2g, Protein 8.3g, Fat 9.1g, Sugar 8.8g, Sodium 1161mg.

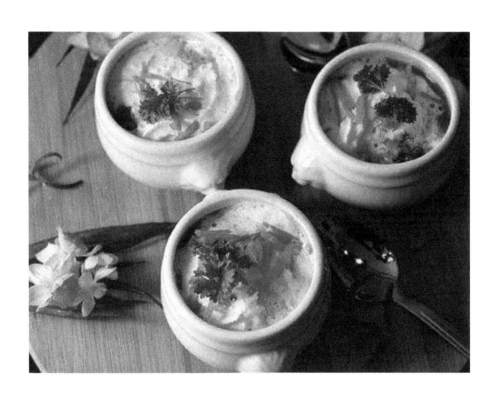

Pork and Mushroom Stew

Preparation Time: 5 Minutes | Cooking Time: 55 Minutes | Servings:6

Ingredients:

2 ½ pounds Pork Cheeks, cut into pieces

1 ½ cups Homemade Chicken Broth

1 Onion, diced

2 tsp minced Garlic

Juice of 1 Lemon

8 ounces Mushrooms, sliced

2 tbsp Olive Oil

1 Leek, sliced

Directions:

Set your Pressure Pot t SAUTE and add the oil to it.

When hot, add the meat and brown it on all sides.

Transfer the meat to a plate and add the onions and leeks. Cook for 3 minutes.

Stir in the garlic and cook for an additional minute.

Return the meat to the pot and place all of the other ingredients inside.

Stir to combine and close the lid.

Cook on MEAT/STEW for 45 minutes.

Do a quick pressure release and open the lid.

Serve immediately and enjoy!

Nutrition:

Calories 510, Total Fats 16g, Carbs 6g, Protein 52g, Dietary Fiber 1.5g.

Thai Chicken

Preparation Time: 10 minutes | Cooking Time: 20 minutes | Servings: 4

Ingredients:

1 lb chicken thighs

For marinade:

1/4 cup creamy peanut butter

1/2 cup hot water

1 tsp ginger, minced

1 tsp garlic, minced

2 tbsp lime juice

2 tbsp sweet chili sauce

1 tbsp soy sauce

1 tbsp sriracha sauce

1/2 tsp salt

Directions:

In a mixing bowl, add all marinade ingredients and whisk until smooth.

Add chicken into the marinade and coat well and place it in the refrigerator overnight.

Place the dehydrating tray in a multi-level air fryer basket and place basket in the Pressure Pot.

Arrange marinated chicken thighs on a dehydrating tray.

Seal pot with air fryer lid and select air fry mode then set the temperature to 350 F and timer for 20 minutes. Turn chicken halfway through.

Serve and enjoy.

Nutrition:

Calories 281, Fat 14.2g, Carbohydrates 0.7g, Sugar 0g, Protein 33g, Cholesterol 116mg.

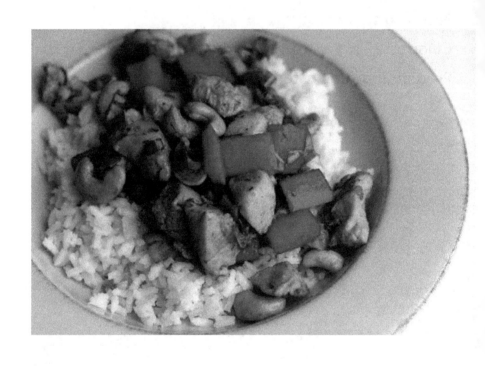

Citrus Herb Chicken

Preparation Time: 10 minutes | Cooking Time: 10 minutes | Servings: 2

Ingredients:

2 chicken breasts, boneless and skinless

1 tsp dried thyme

1 tsp dried oregano

1 tsp dried basil

1 tsp orange zest, grated

1 tsp lemon zest, grated

2 tsp garlic, minced

Pepper

Salt

Directions:

Mix thyme, oregano, basil, orange zest, lemon zest, garlic, pepper, and salt and rub over chicken breasts.

Place the dehydrating tray in a multi-level air fryer basket and place basket in the Pressure Pot.

Place chicken breast on dehydrating tray.

Seal pot with air fryer lid and select air fry mode then set the temperature to 400° F and timer for 10 minutes.

Turn chicken halfway through.

Serve and enjoy.

Nutrition:

Calories 281, Fat 14.2g, Carbohydrates 0.7g, Sugar 0g, Protein 33g, Cholesterol 116mg.

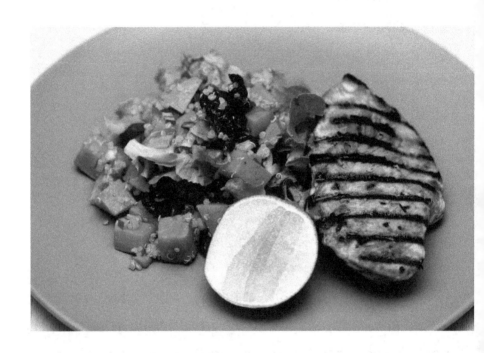

Crispy Crusted Chicken

Preparation Time: 10 minutes | Cooking Time: 14 minutes | Servings: 2

Ingredients:

2 chicken breasts, boneless and skinless

1 tbsp olive oil

2 cups crushed crackers

Pepper

Salt

Directions:

Season chicken with pepper and salt.

Coat chicken with olive oil and coat with crushed crackers.

Place the dehydrating tray in a multi-level air fryer basket and place basket in the Pressure Pot. Place chicken breasts on a dehydrating tray.

Seal pot with air fryer lid and select air fry mode then set the temperature to 370° F and timer for 14 minutes. Turn chicken halfway through.

Serve and enjoy.

Nutrition:

Calories 281, Fat 14.2g, Carbohydrates 0.7g, Sugar 0g, Protein 33g, Cholesterol 116mg.

Italian Chicken Breast

Preparation Time: 10 minutes | Cooking Time: 14 minutes | Servings: 2

Ingredients:

2 chicken breasts, boneless and skinless

8 oz Italian salad dressing

Directions:

Add chicken into the mixing bowl. Pour dressing over chicken and coat well and place in the refrigerator for 1 hour.

Place the dehydrating tray in a multi-level air fryer basket and place basket in the Pressure Pot. Place marinated chicken breasts on a dehydrating tray.

Seal pot with air fryer lid and select air fry mode then set the temperature to 370° F and timer for 14 minutes. Turn chicken halfway through.

Serve and enjoy.

Nutrition:

Calories 281, Fat 14.2g, Carbs 0.7g, Sugar 0g, Protein 33g, Cholesterol 116mg.

Low-Carb Meatloaf

Preparation Time: 10 minutes | Cooking Time: 20 minutes | Servings: 4

Ingredients:

1 egg

1 lb ground beef

1 tbsp garlic powder

1 tsp onion powder

1 1/2 tbsp Worcestershire sauce

2 tbsp tomato paste

1/4 cup half and half

1/4 cup almond flour

Pepper

Salt

Directions:

Spray a loaf pan with cooking spray and set aside.

Add all ingredients into the mixing bowl and mix until well combined.

Transfer meat mixture into the prepared loaf pan.

Place steam rack into the Pressure Pot then places loaf pan on top of the rack.

Seal pot with air fryer lid and select bake mode then set the temperature to 350° F and timer for 20 minutes.

Serve and enjoy.

Nutrition:

Calories 309, Fat 13.3g, Carbohydrates 6.9g, Sugar 2.9g, Protein 38.5g, Cholesterol 148mg.

Indian Meatloaf

Preparation Time: 10 minutes | Cooking Time: 15 minutes | Servings: 4

Ingredients:

2 eggs

1 lb ground beef

1/8 tsp ground cardamom

1/2 tsp ground cinnamon

1 tsp cayenne

1 tsp turmeric

2 tsp garam masala

1 tbsp garlic, minced

1/2 tbsp ginger, minced

1/4 cup fresh cilantro, chopped

1 cup onion, minced

Pepper

Salt

Directions:

Spray a loaf pan with cooking spray and set aside.

Add all ingredients into the mixing bowl and mix until well combined.

Transfer meat mixture into the prepared loaf pan.

Place steam rack into the Pressure Pot then places loaf pan on top of the rack.

Seal pot with air fryer lid and select air fry mode then set the temperature to 360° F and timer for 15 minutes. Serve and enjoy.

Nutrition:

Calories 264, Fat 9.5g, Carbohydrates 5g, Sugar 1.5g, Protein 37.8g, Cholesterol 183mg.

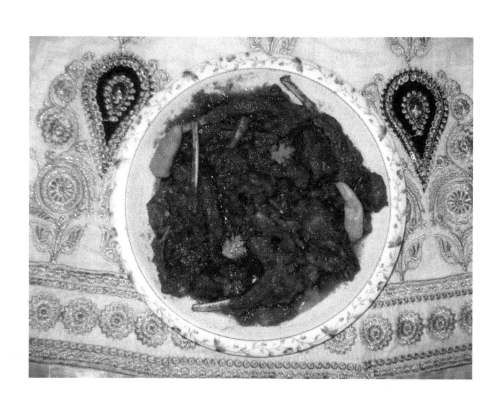

Delicious Kababs

Preparation Time: 10 minutes | Cooking Time: 15 minutes | Servings: 4

Ingredients:

1 lb ground beef

1/4 tsp ground cinnamon

1/4 tsp ground cardamom

1/2 tsp cayenne

1/2 tsp turmeric

1 tbsp ginger, minced

1 tbsp garlic, minced

1/4 cup cilantro, chopped

1/4 cup mint, chopped

1/2 cup onion, minced

1 tsp salt

Directions:

Add meat and remaining ingredients into the mixing bowl and mix until well combined.

Place the dehydrating tray in a multi-level air fryer basket and place basket in the Pressure Pot.

Make kababs into sausage shapes and place them on a dehydrating tray.

Seal pot with air fryer lid and select bake mode then set the temperature to 350° F and timer for 15 minutes. Turn kababs halfway through.

Serve and enjoy.

Nutrition:

Calories 229, Fat 7.3g, Carbohydrates 4g, Sugar 0.7g, Protein 35.1g, Cholesterol 101mg.

Trout and Radishes

Preparation time: 5 minutes | Cooking Time: 12 minutes | Servings: 4

Ingredients:

4 trout fillets, boneless and skinless

A pinch of salt and black pepper

1 tablespoon parsley, chopped

2 tablespoons tomato passata

2 cups red radishes, sliced

Directions:

In your Pressure Pot, combine all the ingredients, put the lid on, and cook on High for 12 minutes.

Release the pressure fast for 5 minutes.

Divide everything between plates and serve.

Nutrition:

Calories 129, fat 5.3g, fiber 1.1g, carbs 2.5g, protein 17g.

Cod and Broccoli

Preparation time: 5 minutes | Cooking Time: 15 minutes | Servings: 4

Ingredients:

4 cod fillets, boneless and skinless

A pinch of salt and black pepper

1-pound broccoli florets

2 tablespoon tomato passata

1 cup chicken stock

1 tablespoon cilantro, chopped

Directions:

In your Pressure Pot, combine all the ingredients, put the lid on, and cook on High for 15 minutes.

Release the pressure fast for 5 minutes, divide the mix between plates and serve.

Nutrition:

Calories 197, fat 10g, fiber 3.1g, carbs 4.3g, protein 19.4g.

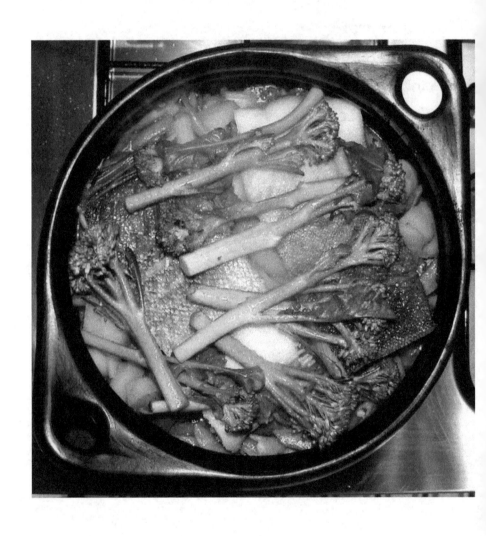

Rosemary Trout and Cauliflower

Preparation time: 10 minutes | Cooking Time: 15 minutes | Servings: 4

Ingredients:

4 trout fillets, boneless and skinless

½ cup veggie stock

2 garlic cloves, minced

2 cups cauliflower florets

1 tablespoon avocado oil

A pinch of salt and black pepper

1 tablespoon rosemary, chopped

Directions:

Set the Pressure Pot on Sauté mode, add the oil, heat it, add the garlic and sauté for 2 minutes.

Add the rest of the ingredients, put the lid on, and cook on High for 13 minutes.

Release the pressure naturally for 10 minutes, divide the mix between plates and serve.

Nutrition:

Calories 140, fat 5.9g, fiber 1.8g, carbs 3.9g, protein 17.7g.

Cinnamon Cod Mix

Preparation time: 5 minutes | Cooking Time: 12 minutes | Servings: 4

Ingredients:

4 cod fillets, boneless and skinless

1 tablespoon cinnamon powder

1 cup cherry tomatoes, cubed

Juice of ½ lemon

½ cup veggie stock

A pinch of salt and black pepper

1 tablespoon cilantro, chopped

Directions:

In your Pressure Pot, mix the fish with the rest of the ingredients, put the lid on and cook on High for 12 minutes.

Release the pressure fast for 5 minutes, divide everything between plates and serve.

Nutrition:

Calories 162, fat 9.6g, fiber 0.3g, carbs 3g, protein 16.5g.

Trout and Eggplant Mix

Preparation time: 10 minutes | Cooking Time: 15 minutes | Servings: 4

Ingredients:

4 trout fillets, boneless

2 scallions, chopped

2 eggplants, cubed

½ cup chicken stock

2 tablespoons parsley, chopped

3 tablespoons olive oil

A pinch of salt and black pepper

2 tablespoons smoked paprika

Directions:

Set the Pressure Pot on Sauté mode, add the oil, heat it, add the scallions and the eggplant and cook for 2 minutes,

Add the rest of the ingredients except the parsley, put the lid on, and cook on High for 13 minutes.

Release the pressure naturally for 10 minutes, divide the mix between plates and serve with the parsley sprinkled on top.

Nutrition:

Calories 291, fat 16.8g, fiber 4.5g, carbs 6.4g, protein 20g.

Salmon and Tomato Passata

Preparation time: 10 minutes | Cooking Time: 15 minutes | Servings: 4

Ingredients:

1 tablespoon olive oil

4 salmon fillets, boneless, skinless, and cubed

1 tablespoon rosemary, chopped

1 shallot, chopped

1 cup tomato passata

1 teaspoon chili powder

1 tablespoon chives, chopped

A pinch of salt and black pepper

Directions:

Set the Pressure Pot on Sauté mode, add the oil, heat it, add the shallot and sauté for 2 minutes.

Add the rest of the ingredients, put the lid on, and cook on High for 12 minutes.

Release the pressure naturally for 10 minutes, divide the mix between plates and serve.

Nutrition:

Calories 291, fat 16.8g, fiber 4.5g, carbs 7.4g, protein 20g.

CPSIA information can be obtained
at www.ICGtesting.com
Printed in the USA
BVHW092104250621
610374BV00006B/960